DYSPHAGIA COOKBOOK FOR NEWLY DIAGNOSED

The Comprehensive Guide to Nourishing and Delicious Soft Food Recipes with a 30-Day Meal Plan for people with Difficulty in Swallowing.

Emily O. Wells

Copyright © 2024 by Emily O. Wells

Thank you for considering this publication. I believe that the "Dysphagia Cookbook for Newly Diagnosed" can make a meaningful difference in the lives of those navigating swallowing anomalies. If you have any questions or would like additional information, please don't hesitate to reach out.

Warm regards,

Emily O. Wells (RDN)

dietwithemillywells@gmail.com

Disclaimer

As an experienced (RDN), I hereby endorse the information's provided in this "Dysphagia Cookbook for Newly Diagnosed" it is intended for general informational purposes and can as well be considered as professional advice.

While the recipes and meal plans are designed to accommodate individuals with dysphagia, it is also crucial to put into cognizance's personalized guidance based on specific underlying medical conditions, dietary needs, and individual tolerances. Thanks

What happened to Joe?

Joe, a vibrant and resilient individual, found himself facing the unexpected challenge of dysphagia. His daily routine was disrupted, and the simple joy of sharing a meal became a daunting task. Determined to regain a sense of normalcy, Joe embarked on a quest for a solution.

He Discovered the "Dysphagia Cookbook for Newly Diagnosed." Skeptical yet hopeful, Joe enter into its pages, discovering a treasure trove of soft food recipes crafted with both nourishment and flavor in mind

The recipes, from velvety breakfast smoothies to savory, easy-to-swallow dinners, not only catered to Joe's nutritional needs but also rekindled his love for the art of dining. Each page turned unveiled a new possibility, a new taste sensation, and, most importantly, a renewed sense of joy around the dinner table.

As the 30-day meal plan unfolded, Joe's confidence grew. The once-feared prospect of meals became a daily celebration of victory over adversity. His journey with this cookbook not only addressed his swallowing anomaly but also created a bridge back to the shared joy of family dinners and gatherings with friends.

In the heartwarming tale of Joe's journey, **"Dysphagia Cookbook for Newly Diagnosed: The Comprehensive Guide to Nourishing and Delicious Soft Food Recipes with a 30-Day Meal Plan for people with Difficulty in Swallowing"** became more than just a collection of recipes. It became a companion, a blueprint, and a testament to the transformative power of adapting and embracing new possibilities. Joe's story is a testament to the cookbook's potential to bring comfort, nourishment, and a renewed zest for life to those navigating the challenges of dysphagia.

TABLE OF CONTENT

CHAPTER 1

ANATOMY OF SWALLOWING

Swallowing is a complex and precisely coordinated process that involves multiple muscles and structures working seamlessly to transport food and liquids from the mouth to the stomach. Understanding the anatomy of swallowing is essential in comprehending the challenges individuals with dysphagia face.

1. Oral Phase:

- **Mouth and Tongue:** The process begins with the manipulation of food by the tongue and the mixing of saliva, forming a cohesive bolus.

- **Soft Palate and Uvula:** These structures prevent food and liquids from entering the nasal cavity during swallowing.

2. Pharyngeal Phase:

- **Pharynx:** The bolus is propelled through the pharynx by a series of muscle contractions.

- **Epiglottis:** This flap-like structure protects the airway by covering the trachea during swallowing, ensuring that food and liquids enter the esophagus.

3. Esophageal Phase:

- **Esophagus:** The bolus travels down the esophagus through peristaltic waves, reaching the lower esophageal sphincter.

- **Lower Esophageal Sphincter:** This muscular ring relaxes to allow the bolus to enter the stomach.

COMMON CAUSES OF DYSPHAGIA

Dysphagia, or difficulty swallowing, can result from various underlying conditions affecting different stages of the swallowing process. Common causes include:

1. Neurological Disorders:

- **Stroke:** Damage to the brain regions responsible for swallowing coordination.

- **Parkinson's disease:** Degeneration of nerve cells affecting muscle control.

2. Structural Issues:

- **Esophageal Stricture:** Narrowing of the esophagus due to scarring or inflammation.
- **Tumors:** Growth in the throat or esophagus impeding the passage of food.

3. Muscular Disorders:

- **Achalasia:** Impaired relaxation of the lower esophageal sphincter.

- **Myasthenia Gravis:** Weakness in the muscles involved in swallowing.

4. Gastroesophageal Reflux Disease (GRD): This usually occur when stomach acid repeatedly flows back into the tube connecting your mouth and stomach (esophagus).

TYPES AND STAGES OF DYSPHAGIA

1. Oropharyngeal Dysphagia:

- Affecting the oral and pharyngeal phases.

- Difficulty initiating a swallow, coughing during meals, or experiencing food sticking in the throat.

2. Esophageal Dysphagia:

- Primarily impacting the esophageal phase.

- Sensation of food getting stuck in the chest, pain while swallowing, or regurgitation.

THE DYSPHAGIA DIET

The dysphagia diet is a crucial aspect of managing swallowing difficulties, tailored to the specific needs of individuals. It involves texture modifications to ensure safe and comfortable swallowing:

Level 1: Pureed Diet:

- Blended and smooth consistency suitable for those with severe dysphagia.
- Examples include pureed fruits, vegetables, and meats.

Level 2: Mechanical Soft Diet:

- Soft, moist, and easily chewed textures.
- Cooked fruits, ground or finely diced meats, and soft casseroles.

Level 3: Advanced Diet:

- More varied textures suitable for individuals with mild to moderate dysphagia.
- Tender meats, moist bread, and softer raw fruits and vegetables.

30-DAY SOFT FOOD MEAL PLAN

Embarking on a 30-day soft food journey is an opportunity to infuse variety, nutrition, and flavor into the daily meals of those managing dysphagia. This meticulously crafted meal plan is structured across four weeks, each with its unique theme and culinary exploration.

Week 1: Gentle Beginnings

In the initial week, the focus is on introducing easily digestible and comforting options. The goal is to acclimate the palate to softer textures while providing essential nutrients.

Day 1-7:

- **Breakfast:** Creamy oatmeal with mashed bananas.
- **Lunch:** Pureed vegetable soup and a soft turkey sandwich.
- **Dinner:** Tender chicken stew with well-cooked carrots and peas.

Building on the foundation of the first week, Week 2 introduces a broader spectrum of flavors. Soft doesn't mean bland; it's an invitation to explore the richness of well-seasoned, easily chewable options.

Day 8-14:

- **Breakfast:** Blended berry and yogurt smoothie.
- **Lunch:** Mechanical soft fish tacos with avocado salsa.
- **Dinner:** Soft meatballs with marinara sauce and mashed sweet potatoes.

Week 3:

Week 3 expands the repertoire with diverse culinary experiences. This week aims to celebrate the art of soft cooking with globally inspired and creatively adapted dishes.

Day 15-21:

- **Breakfast:** Soft scrambled eggs with spinach and feta.
- **Lunch:** Pureed lentil curry with soft naan bread. (Flatbread)
- **Dinner:** Shredded soft chicken tacos with lime and cilantro.

Week 4:

As the journey reaches its culmination, Week 4 combines the lessons learned from the previous weeks, creating a symphony of tastes and textures.

Day 22-30:

- **Breakfast:** Banana and almond butter smoothie bowl.
- **Lunch:** Soft chicken Caesar salad with avocado.
- **Dinner:** Slow-cooked pot roast with mashed cauliflower.

CHAPTER 2

BREAKFAST FOR SWALLOWING EASE

1. Smoothies and Shakes

a. Berry Bliss Smoothie:

Ingredients:

- 1 cup mixed berries (strawberries, blueberries, raspberries)
- 1/2 cup yogurt (Greek or regular)
- 1 banana, peeled and sliced
- 1/2 cup almond milk
- 1 tablespoon honey (optional)

Preparation:

1. Blend berries, yogurt, banana, and almond milk until smooth.
2. Add honey for sweetness if desired.
3. Serve chilled.

b. Green Power Protein Smoothie:

Ingredients:

- 1 cup spinach leaves
- 1/2 cup cucumber, peeled and chopped
- 1/2 avocado, peeled and pitted
- 1/2 cup plain yogurt
- 1/2 cup water or coconut water

Preparation:

1. Blend spinach, cucumber, avocado, yogurt, and water until smooth.
2. Adjust thickness by adding more water if needed.
3. Pour into a glass and enjoy.

2. Porridge and Oatmeal Creations

a. Apple Cinnamon Quinoa Porridge:

Ingredients:

- 1/2 cup quinoa, rinsed

- 1 cup almond milk

- 1 apple, peeled, cored, and diced

- 1/2 teaspoon cinnamon

- 1 tablespoon maple syrup

Preparation:

1. Combine quinoa and almond milk in a saucepan.

2. Cook over medium heat until quinoa is tender and liquid is absorbed.

3. Stir in diced apples, cinnamon, and maple syrup.

4. Cook for an additional 2-3 minutes, stirring occasionally.

b. Nutty Banana Quinoa Porridge:

Ingredients:

- 1/2 cup quinoa, rinsed

- 1 cup coconut milk

- 1 banana, mashed

- 2 tablespoons chopped nuts (almonds, walnuts)

- 1 tablespoon honey

Preparation:

1. Cook quinoa in coconut milk until tender.
2. Stir in mashed banana, chopped nuts, and honey.
3. Cook for an additional 2 minutes, ensuring a creamy consistency.

3. Soft Breakfast Casseroles

a. Spinach and Feta Egg Casserole:

Ingredients:

- 4 eggs
- 1 cup spinach, chopped
- 1/2 cup feta cheese, crumbled
- 1/4 cup milk
- Salt and pepper to taste

Preparation:

1. Whisk eggs, milk, salt, and pepper together.
2. Stir in chopped spinach and feta.
3. Pour into a greased baking dish and bake until set.

b. Sausage and Mushroom Breakfast Bake:

Ingredients:

- 1/2 cup cooked sausage, crumbled
- 1/2 cup mushrooms, sliced
- 4 eggs
- 1/4 cup milk
- Salt and pepper to taste

Preparation:

1. Combine cooked sausage and mushrooms in a baking dish.
2. Whisk eggs, milk, salt, and pepper together.
3. Pour over the sausage and mushrooms, bake until eggs are set.

4. Creamy Banana Almond Smoothie:

Ingredients:

- 1 ripe banana
- 1/2 cup Greek yogurt
- 1/4 cup almond milk
- 1 tablespoon almond butter

Preparation:

1. Blend banana, Greek yogurt, almond milk, and almond butter until smooth.
2. Adjust thickness by adding more almond milk if needed.
3. Serve in a dysphagia-friendly consistency.

5. Soft Scrambled Eggs with Spinach:

Ingredients:

- 2 eggs
- 1/4 cup cooked and chopped spinach
- Salt and pepper to taste

Preparation:

1. Whisk eggs and cook gently in a non-stick pan.

2. Stir in cooked spinach, season with salt and pepper.

3. Ensure a soft, easily chewable texture.

6. Pumpkin Spice Oatmeal Mash:

Ingredients:

- 1/2 cup instant oats
- 1/2 cup pumpkin puree
- 1 tablespoon honey

Preparation:

1. Cook instant oats as per package instructions.

2. Stir in pumpkin puree and honey.

3. Mash for a soft consistency.

7. Avocado and Cottage Cheese Mash:

Ingredients:

- 1/2 ripe avocado
- 1/2 cup cottage cheese

- A pinch of salt

Preparation:

1. Mash avocado and mix with cottage cheese.
2. Add a pinch of salt for flavor.
3. Ensure a smooth and soft texture.

8. Soft Blueberry Pancakes:

Ingredients:

1/2 cup pancake mix (dysphagia-friendly)

1/4 cup mashed blueberries

1/4 cup milk

Preparation:

Mix pancake mix with mashed blueberries and milk.

Cook on a griddle until soft and fluffy.

Serve in small, easily manageable portions.

9. Mango Yogurt Parfait:

Ingredients:

- 1/2 cup diced mango
- 1/2 cup yogurt
- 2 tablespoons granola (blended for softness)

Preparation:

1. Layer diced mango, yogurt, and blended granola.
2. Repeat layers for a visually appealing and tasty parfait.

10. Soft French toast Bites:

Ingredients:

- 1 slice dysphagia-friendly bread
- 1 egg
- 1/4 cup milk

Preparation:

1. Cut dysphagia-friendly bread into bite-sized pieces.

2. Whisk egg and milk, soak bread bites, then cook until soft.

11. Chia Seed Pudding with Berries:

Ingredients:

- 2 tablespoons chia seeds
- 1/2 cup almond milk
- Mixed berries for topping

Preparation:

1. Mix chia seeds with almond milk, let it sit until thickened.
2. Top with mixed berries for added flavor and nutrition.

12. Applesauce and Cinnamon Quinoa:

Ingredients:

- 1/2 cup cooked quinoa
- 1/4 cup applesauce
- A dash of cinnamon

Preparation:

1. Mix cooked quinoa with applesauce and cinnamon.
2. Ensure a soft and easily swallow able consistency.

13. Soft Breakfast Casserole:

Ingredients:

- 2 eggs
- 1/4 cup cooked and mashed sweet potato
- 1 tablespoon shredded cheese

Preparation:

1. Whisk eggs and mix with mashed sweet potato.
2. Pour into a greased dish, sprinkle with cheese, and bake until set.

14. Mango Coconut Chia Parfait:

Ingredients:

- 2 tablespoons chia seeds
- 1/2 cup mango, diced
- 1/4 cup coconut milk

Preparation:

1. Layer chia seeds, diced mango, and coconut milk in a glass.

15. Soft Cheese and Tomato Wrap:

Ingredients:

- 1 soft tortilla
- 2 tablespoons cream cheese
- 1/2 tomato, sliced

Preparation:

1. Spread cream cheese on the tortilla.
2. Add sliced tomatoes and roll into a wrap.

CHAPTER 3

SATISFYING LUNCHES FOR DYSPHAGIA WELLNESS

1. Chicken and Rice Congee:

Ingredients:

- 1/2 cup cooked rice
- 1/2 cup shredded chicken
- 1 cup chicken broth
- 1 tablespoon chopped green onions

Preparation:

1. Simmer cooked rice, shredded chicken, and chicken broth until well blended.
2. Garnish with chopped green onions.

2. Creamy Potato Leek Soup:

Ingredients:

- 1 cup potatoes, peeled and diced
- 1/2 cup leeks, chopped
- 1 cup vegetable broth
- 2 tablespoons cream

Preparation:

1. Cook potatoes and leeks in vegetable broth until tender.
2. Blend until smooth, then stir in cream.

3. Soft Tofu and Vegetable Stir-Fry:

Ingredients:

- 1/2 cup soft tofu, cubed
- 1/2 cup mixed vegetables (carrots, peas, and broccoli)
- 1 tablespoon soy sauce
- 1 teaspoon sesame oil

Preparation:

1. Sauté soft tofu and mixed vegetables in sesame oil.

2. Add soy sauce and stir until well-cooked.

4. Mashed Sweet Potato and Turkey Casserole:

Ingredients:

- 1/2 cup mashed sweet potatoes
- 1/2 cup ground turkey, cooked
- 1/4 cup turkey gravy
- 1 tablespoon chopped parsley

Preparation:

1. Layer mashed sweet potatoes and cooked ground turkey in a casserole dish.
2. Pour turkey gravy over the layers and bake until heated through.

5. Salmon and Avocado Soft Wrap:

Ingredients:

- 1 soft tortilla
- 1/2 cup canned salmon, flaked
- 1/4 avocado, mashed
- Lettuce leaves

Preparation:

- Spread mashed avocado on the soft tortilla.
- Add flaked salmon and lettuce, then wrap.

6. Lentil and Spinach Puree:

Ingredients:

1. 1/2 cup cooked lentils
2. 1/2 cup cooked spinach
3. 1/4 cup vegetable broth
4. 1 teaspoon olive oil

Preparation:

1. Blend cooked lentils and spinach with vegetable broth until smooth.
2. Drizzle with olive oil before serving.

7. Soft Chicken and Vegetable Stew:

Ingredients:

1/2 cup shredded cooked chicken

1/2 cup mixed vegetables (carrots, peas, corn)

1 cup chicken broth

1 tablespoon fresh herbs (parsley, thyme)

Preparation:

Simmer shredded chicken and mixed vegetables in chicken broth until tender.

Garnish with fresh herbs.

8. Creamy Mushroom and Polenta:

Ingredients:

- 1/2 cup sliced mushrooms
- 1/2 cup soft polenta
- 1/4 cup vegetable broth
- 1 tablespoon cream

Preparation:

1. Sauté mushrooms, then mix with soft polenta and vegetable broth.
2. Stir in cream for a creamy consistency.

9. Quinoa and Black Bean Mash:

Ingredients:

- 1/2 cup cooked quinoa
- 1/2 cup black beans, mashed
- 1/4 cup salsa
- 1 tablespoon cilantro, chopped

Preparation:

1. Combine cooked quinoa and mashed black beans.
2. Top with salsa and chopped cilantro.

10. Spinach and Feta Egg Custard:

Ingredients:

1. 2 eggs, beaten
2. 1/2 cup cooked and chopped spinach
3. 1/4 cup feta cheese, crumbled
4. Salt and pepper to taste

Preparation:

1. Mix beaten eggs with cooked spinach, feta, salt, and pepper.
2. Bake until set to create a custard.

11. Turkey and Cranberry Soft Sandwich:

Ingredients:

1. 1 slice soft bread

2. 1/2 cup sliced turkey

3. 2 tablespoons cranberry sauce

4. Lettuce leaves

Preparation:

1. Layer sliced turkey and cranberry sauce on soft bread.

2. Add lettuce leaves and assemble into a sandwich.

12. Soft Bean and Cheese Quesadilla:

Ingredients:

- 1 soft tortilla
- 1/2 cup black beans, mashed
- 1/4 cup shredded cheese
- Salsa for dipping

Preparation:

1. Spread mashed black beans and shredded cheese on the soft tortilla.

2. Fold in half and heat until cheese melts. Serve with salsa.

13. Shrimp and Avocado Puree:

Ingredients:

- 1/2 cup cooked and mashed shrimp
- 1/2 avocado, mashed
- 1 tablespoon lime juice
- Fresh cilantro for garnish

Preparation:

1. Mix mashed shrimp with mashed avocado.
2. Drizzle with lime juice and garnish with fresh cilantro.

14. Soft Chicken and Rice Bowl:

Ingredients:

- 1/2 cup shredded cooked chicken
- 1/2 cup cooked rice
- 1/4 cup chicken broth

- 1 tablespoon chopped scallions

Preparation:

1. Combine shredded chicken and cooked rice.

2. Pour chicken broth over the mixture and top with chopped scallions.

15. Hummus and Roasted Vegetable Wrap:

Ingredients:

- 1 soft tortilla

- 2 tablespoons hummus

- 1/2 cup roasted vegetables (bell peppers, zucchini)

- Fresh herbs for garnish

Preparation:

1. Spread hummus on the soft tortilla.

2. Add roasted vegetables and garnish with fresh herbs before rolling into a wrap.

CHAPTER 4

DINNER FOR DYSPHAGIA WELLNESS

1. Creamy Chicken and Rice Casserole:

Ingredients:

- 1 cup shredded cooked chicken
- 1/2 cup cooked rice
- 1/2 cup mixed vegetables (peas, carrots)
- 1/2 cup chicken broth
- 2 tablespoons cream

Instructions:

1. Combine shredded chicken, cooked rice, mixed vegetables, chicken broth, and cream.
2. Bake until bubbly and golden.

2. Soft Baked Cod with Mashed Sweet Potatoes:

Ingredients:

- 1 cod fillet, baked until flaky

- 1/2 cup mashed sweet potatoes

- 1 tablespoon olive oil

- Fresh parsley for garnish

Instructions:

1. Bake the cod fillet until it easily flakes with a fork.

2. Serve over mashed sweet potatoes, drizzle with olive oil, and garnish with fresh parsley.

3. Quinoa and Vegetable Stir-Fry:

Ingredients:

- 1/2 cup cooked quinoa

- 1/2 cup mixed stir-fry vegetables (broccoli, bell peppers)

- 1 tablespoon soy sauce

- 1 teaspoon sesame oil

Instructions:

1. Sauté cooked quinoa and mixed vegetables in sesame oil.

2. Add soy sauce and stir until well-cooked.

4. Tender Turkey Meatballs with Tomato Sauce:

Ingredients:

- 1/2 cup ground turkey formed into meatballs
- 1/2 cup tomato sauce
- 1/4 cup grated Parmesan cheese
- Fresh basil for garnish

Instructions:

1. Cook turkey meatballs until fully cooked.

2. Serve with tomato sauce, sprinkle with Parmesan cheese, and garnish with fresh basil.

5. Creamy Butternut Squash Soup:

Ingredients:

- 1 cup butternut squash, cooked and pureed
- 1/2 cup vegetable broth
- 2 tablespoons cream
- Ground nutmeg for seasoning

Instructions:

1. Blend cooked butternut squash with vegetable broth and cream.
2. Season with ground nutmeg to taste.

6. Soft Beef and Vegetable Stew:

Ingredients:

- 1/2 cup shredded cooked beef
- 1/2 cup mixed stew vegetables (carrots, potatoes)
- 1 cup beef broth
- 1 tablespoon tomato paste

Instructions:

1. Simmer shredded beef and mixed vegetables in beef broth.
2. Stir in tomato paste until well-combined.

7. Salmon and Avocado Mash:

Ingredients:

- 1 salmon fillet, baked until flaky
- 1/2 avocado, mashed
- 1 tablespoon lemon juice
- Fresh dill for garnish

Instructions:

1. Bake the salmon fillet until it easily flakes.
2. Mash avocado, mix with lemon juice, and garnish with fresh dill.

8. Lentil and Carrot Puree:

Ingredients:

- 1/2 cup cooked lentils
- 1/2 cup cooked and pureed carrots
- 1/4 cup vegetable broth
- 1 teaspoon olive oil

Instructions:

1. Blend cooked lentils, carrot puree, vegetable broth, and olive oil until smooth.
2. Adjust consistency as needed.

9. Soft Eggplant and Tomato Bake:

Ingredients:

- 1 cup eggplant, baked until soft
- 1/2 cup tomato sauce
- 1/4 cup mozzarella cheese, shredded
- Fresh basil for garnish

Instructions:

1. Bake eggplant until soft, then layer with tomato sauce and mozzarella.
2. Bake until cheese is melted, and garnish with fresh basil.

10. Creamy Spinach and Feta Risotto:

Ingredients:

- 1/2 cup Arborio rice, cooked
- 1/2 cup cooked and chopped spinach
- 1/4 cup feta cheese, crumbled
- 1/4 cup vegetable broth

Instructions:

1. Combine cooked rice, spinach, feta, and vegetable broth.
2. Stir until well-mixed and creamy.

11. Soft Chicken and Broccoli Alfredo:

Ingredients:

- 1/2 cup shredded cooked chicken
- 1/2 cup steamed broccoli florets
- 1/2 cup Alfredo sauce
- Cooked pasta of choice

Instructions:

1. Mix shredded chicken and steamed broccoli with Alfredo sauce.
2. Serve over cooked pasta.

12. Quinoa and Black Bean Stuffed Peppers:

Ingredients:

1. 1/2 cup cooked quinoa
2. 1/2 cup black beans, mashed
3. 1/4 cup salsa
4. Bell peppers, halved and roasted

Instructions:

1. Combine cooked quinoa, mashed black beans, and salsa.
2. Stuff the mixture into roasted bell peppers.

13. Soft Tofu and Mushroom Stir-Fry:

Ingredients:

- 1/2 cup soft tofu, cubed
- 1/2 cup sliced mushrooms
- 1/4 cup soy sauce
- 1 tablespoon sesame oil

Instructions:

1. Sauté soft tofu and sliced mushrooms in sesame oil.
2. Add soy sauce and stir until well-cooked.

14. Turkey and Cranberry Soft Casserole:

Ingredients:

- 1/2 cup ground turkey, cooked
- 1/2 cup cranberry sauce
- 1/4 cup breadcrumbs
- 1 tablespoon melted butter

Instructions:

1. Mix cooked ground turkey with cranberry sauce.
2. Top with breadcrumbs mixed with melted butter and bake until golden.

15. Soft Polenta with Roasted Vegetables:

Ingredients:

- 1/2 cup soft polenta
- 1/2 cup roasted vegetables (zucchini, cherry tomatoes)
- 1/4 cup grated Parmesan cheese
- Fresh basil for garnish

Instructions:

Serve soft polenta with roasted vegetables.

Sprinkle with grated Parmesan and garnish with fresh basil.

CHAPTER 5

EASY TO SWALLOW SNACKS

1. Avocado and Banana Smoothie:

Ingredients:

- 1/2 avocado, mashed
- 1 ripe banana
- 1/2 cup yogurt
- Honey for sweetness (optional)

Preparation:

1. Blend mashed avocado, banana, and yogurt until smooth.
2. Add honey if desired and blend again.

2. Soft Apple Slices with Peanut Butter:

Ingredients:

- Softened apple slices
- Peanut butter

Preparation:

1. Spread a thin layer of peanut butter on softened apple slices.

3. Greek Yogurt and Berry Parfait:

Ingredients:

- Greek yogurt
- Mixed berries (blueberries, strawberries)
- Granola for texture (optional)

Preparation:

2. Layer Greek yogurt with mixed berries in a glass.
3. Add granola for extra crunch if desired.

4. Cottage Cheese with Soft Mango Cubes:

Ingredients:

- Cottage cheese
- Ripe mango, cubed

Preparation:

1. Combine cottage cheese with soft mango cubes.

5. Hummus and Soft Pita Bread:

Ingredients:

- Hummus
- Soft pita bread, cut into small pieces

Preparation:

1. Dip soft pita bread into hummus for a satisfying snack.

6. Mashed Banana and Walnut Bites:

Ingredients:

- Mashed banana
- Chopped walnuts

Preparation:

2. Mix mashed banana with chopped walnuts.

3. Form into bite-sized portions.

7. Chilled Cucumber and Yogurt Soup:

Ingredients:

- Blended cucumber
- Yogurt
- Fresh dill for flavor

Preparation:

1. Blend cucumber and yogurt until smooth.
2. Garnish with fresh dill.

8. Soft Cheese and Grapes:

Ingredients:

- Soft cheese (brie, camembert)
- Seedless grapes

Preparation:

1. Pair soft cheese with grapes for a delightful combination.

9. Pear and Cottage Cheese Cup:

Ingredients:

- Softened pear, diced
- Cottage cheese

Preparation:

2. Mix diced pear with cottage cheese.

10. Oatmeal Cookie Bites:

Ingredients:

- Soft oatmeal cookies, crumbled
- Greek yogurt

Preparation:

2. Top Greek yogurt with crumbled oatmeal cookies.

11. Soft Boiled Egg and Toast Soldiers:

Ingredients:

Soft boiled egg

Softened toast, cut into soldiers

Preparation:

Dip softened toast soldiers into a soft-boiled egg.

12. Blended Watermelon Slush:

Ingredients:

- Blended watermelon
- Ice cubes

Preparation:

3. Blend watermelon into a refreshing slush.

13. Peanut Butter and Banana Soft Wrap:

Ingredients:

- Soft tortilla
- Peanut butter
- Sliced banana

Preparation:

1. Spread peanut butter on a soft tortilla, add sliced banana, and wrap.

14. Soft Rice Pudding Cups:

Ingredients:

- Soft rice pudding
- Cinnamon for flavor

Preparation:

1. Sprinkle cinnamon on top of soft rice pudding.

15. Peach and Yogurt Smoothie Bowl:

Ingredients:

- Blended ripe peach
- Yogurt
- Granola for texture

Preparation:

1. Pour blended peach over a bowl of yogurt and top with granola.

CHAPTER 6

EASY-TO-SWALLOW TREATS

Ensuring treats are easy to swallow is crucial for individuals managing dysphagia.

1. Soft Chocolate Mousse:

Ingredients:

- 1 cup chocolate pudding
- 1/2 cup whipped cream

Instructions:

1. Gently fold whipped cream into chocolate pudding.
2. Chill before serving.

2. Chilled Banana Popsicles:

Ingredients:

- Blended ripe bananas
- Coconut milk

Instructions Mix blended bananas with coconut milk.

1. Pour into popsicle molds and freeze.

3. Berry Yogurt Bites:

Ingredients:

- Mixed berry yogurt
- Gelatin

Instructions:

1. Mix gelatin into berry yogurt.
2. Set in molds and refrigerate until firm.

4. Applesauce and Cinnamon Cups:

Ingredients:

Unsweetened applesauce

Ground cinnamon

Instructions:

Sprinkle ground cinnamon on top of applesauce.

5. Soft Mango Sorbet:

Ingredients:

- Blended ripe mango
- Lemon juice

Instructions:

1. Blend mango with lemon juice.
2. Freeze until a sorbet consistency is achieved.

6. Pudding Parfait with Berries:

Ingredients:

- Vanilla pudding
- Mixed berries

Instructions:

1. Layer vanilla pudding with mixed berries in a cup.

7. Mashed Sweet Potato Bites:

Ingredients:

- Mashed sweet potatoes

- Maple syrup

Instructions:

2. Form mashed sweet potatoes into bite-sized portions.
3. Drizzle with maple syrup.

8. Soft Lemon Squares:

Ingredients:

- Soft lemon squares
- Powdered sugar for dusting

Instructions:

1. Dust soft lemon squares with powdered sugar.

9. Whipped Cream and Peach Cups:

Ingredients:

- Whipped cream
- Softened canned peaches

Instructions:

1. Layer whipped cream with softened peaches in cups.

10. Creamy Avocado Popsicles:

Ingredients:

- Blended ripe avocado
- Condensed milk

Instructions:

1. Blend avocado with condensed milk.
2. Pour into popsicle molds and freeze.

11. Nut Butter Banana Bites:

Ingredients:

1. Sliced ripe banana
2. Almond butter or peanut butter

Instructions:

1. Spread nut butter on banana slices.

12. Soft Pumpkin Pie Cups:

Ingredients:

1. Soft pumpkin pie filling
2. Whipped cream

Instructions:

1. Spoon soft pumpkin pie filling into cups.
2. Top with whipped cream.

13. Mixed Fruit Gel Cups:

Ingredients:

- Fruit-flavored gelatin
- Mixed canned fruit in juice

Instructions:

1. Prepare fruit-flavored gelatin as directed.
2. Mix in canned fruit and let it set.

14. Soft Blueberry Cheesecake Bites:

Ingredients:

- Soft blueberry cheesecake
- Fresh blueberries for garnish

Instructions:

1. Cut soft blueberry cheesecake into bite-sized pieces.
2. Garnish with fresh blueberries.

15. Honeyed Yogurt Drops:

Ingredients:

- Greek yogurt
- Honey

Instructions:

1. Mix honey into Greek yogurt.
2. Drop small portions onto a parchment-lined tray and freeze.

CHAPTER 7

BEVERAGES FOR EASY SWALLOWING

Ensuring beverages are easy to swallow is essential for individuals managing dysphagia. Here are 15 refreshing and easy-to-swallow beverages with detailed instructions:

1. Chilled Cucumber Mint Smoothie:

Ingredients:

- Blended cucumber
- Fresh mint leaves
- Ice cubes

Instructions:

1. Blend cucumber and mint until smooth.
2. Serve over ice.

2. Watermelon Slush:

Ingredients:

- Blended watermelon

- Ice cubes

Instructions:

1. Blend watermelon until slushy.
2. Pour into a chilled glass.

3. Lemon Ginger Infused Water:

Ingredients:

- Lemon slices
- Fresh ginger, thinly sliced
- Water

Instructions:

1. Infuse lemon slices and ginger in water.
2. Chill before serving.

4. Apple Juice with a Hint of Cinnamon:

Ingredients:

- Unsweetened apple juice
- Ground cinnamon

Instructions:

1. Mix ground cinnamon into apple juice.
2. Serve chilled.

5. Coconut Water with Pineapple Essence:

Ingredients:

- Coconut water
- Pineapple essence

Instructions:

1. Add a few drops of pineapple essence to coconut water.
2. Chill and enjoy.

6. Mashed Banana Smoothie:

Ingredients:

- Mashed ripe banana
- Yogurt
- Honey for sweetness (optional)

Instructions:

1. Blend mashed banana and yogurt until smooth.

2. Add honey if desired.

7. Soft Berry Tea:

Ingredients:

- Berry herbal tea
- Honey for sweetness (optional)

Instructions:

1. Brew berry herbal tea and let it cool.
2. Add honey if desired.

8. Peach Nectar Spritzer:

Ingredients:

- Peach nectar
- Sparkling water

Instructions:

1. Mix peach nectar with sparkling water.
2. Serve over ice.

9. Avocado and Spinach Smoothie:

Ingredients:

- Blended ripe avocado
- Fresh spinach leaves
- Coconut milk

Instructions:

1. Blend avocado, spinach, and coconut milk until smooth.
2. Chill before serving.

10. Chilled Blueberry Lemonade:

Ingredients:

- Blueberry juice
- Freshly squeezed lemon juice
- Ice cubes

Instructions:

1. Mix blueberry juice with freshly squeezed lemon juice.
2. Serve over ice.

11. Creamy Vanilla Milkshake:

Ingredients:

- Vanilla ice cream
- Milk

Instructions:

1. Blend vanilla ice cream with milk until creamy.
2. Serve chilled.

12. Carrot and Orange Smoothie:

Ingredients:

- Blended carrots
- Freshly squeezed orange juice
- Ice cubes

Instructions:

1. Blend carrots and orange juice until smooth.
2. Serve over ice.

13. Minty Honeydew Cooler:

Ingredients:

- Blended honeydew melon
- Fresh mint leaves
- Sparkling water

Instructions:

1. Blend honeydew melon and mint until smooth.
2. Mix with sparkling water.

14. Raspberry Almond Milkshake:

Ingredients:

- Frozen raspberries
- Almond milk
- Honey for sweetness (optional)

Instructions:

1. Blend frozen raspberries and almond milk until smooth.
2. Add honey if desired.

15. Warm Vanilla Almond Milk:

Ingredients:

- Warmed almond milk
- Vanilla extract
- Cinnamon for flavor

Instructions:

1. Warm almond milk and mix in vanilla extract.
2. Sprinkle with cinnamon.

Appendix:

Dysphagia-Friendly Ingredients Index

This index lists key elements that cater to individuals managing swallowing difficulties and acts as a valuable tool for selecting, planning, and creating meals that prioritize both nutrition and ease of swallowing

Common Ingredients:

1. Soft Fruits (e.g., ripe bananas, peaches, and avocados)
2. Mashed Vegetables (e.g., sweet potatoes, carrots)
3. Soft Proteins (e.g., shredded chicken, tofu)
4. Gelatin for Creating Soft Desserts
5. Nut Butters (e.g., almond butter, peanut butter)
6. Dairy Alternatives (e.g., almond milk, coconut milk)
7. Unsweetened Applesauce
8. Soft Grains (e.g., oatmeal, rice pudding)
9. Puddings and Custards
10. Soft Breads and Tortillas

Flavor Enhancers:

1. Mild Herbs (e.g., parsley, chives)
2. Ground Spices (e.g., cinnamon, ginger)
3. Lemon Juice for Zest
4. Vanilla Extract for Sweet Treats
5. Soft Cheese Varieties
6. Honey for Natural Sweetness
7. Berry Extracts for Flavorful Options

Beverage Additions:

1. Coconut Water for Hydration
2. Flavored Herbal Teas
3. Fruit Juices without Pulp
4. Sparkling Water for Effervescence

Glossary of Terms

1. **Aspiration:** Inhaling food or liquid into the airways, which can lead to respiratory issues

2. **Bolus:** A cohesive mass of food prepared for swallowing.

3. **Cricopharyngeal Muscle:** The muscle responsible for opening and closing the upper esophageal sphincter during swallowing.

4. **Dysphagia:** Difficulty or discomfort in swallowing, often caused by various medical conditions.

5. **Enteral Nutrition**: Providing nutrients directly into the digestive tract, often through a feeding tube.

6. **Fiber:** Plant-based material that aids in digestion and supports gut health.

7. **Gastroesophageal Reflux Disease (GERD):** Chronic digestive disorder causing stomach acid to flow back into the esophagus.

8. **Gelatin:** A thickening agent often used in dysphagia-friendly desserts.

9. **Hydration:** Maintaining adequate fluid levels in the body.

10. **Irrigation:** Cleaning and flushing a feeding tube to prevent clogs.

11. **J-Tube:** Jejunostomy tube, a feeding tube inserted directly into the jejunum.

12. **Kosher:** Food prepared according to Jewish dietary laws.

13. **Larynx:** The voice box, containing the vocal cords.

14. **Mastication:** The process of chewing food.

15. **Nectar-Thick:** A consistency level for liquids used in dysphagia management.

16. **Oropharynx:** The middle part of the throat.

17. **Puree:** Food blended to a smooth, creamy consistency.

18. **Quadriplegia:** Paralysis affecting all four limbs.

19. **Regurgitation:** The backward flow of stomach contents into the mouth.

20. **Soft Diet:** A diet consisting of foods that are easy to chew and swallow.

21. **Tracheotomy:** Surgical procedure creating an opening in the windpipe to assist breathing.

22. **Umami:** A savory taste often associated with broths and cooked meats.

23. **Ventilator:** A machine assisting with breathing, often used in critical care.

24. **Whole Grains**: Grains that retain all parts of the seed, providing more nutrients.

25. **Xanthan Gum:** A thickening agent used in dysphagia-friendly recipes.

26. **Yogurt:** A dairy product containing beneficial bacteria for gut health.

27. **Zenker's Diverticulum:** A pouch that can form in the wall of the throat.

28. **Al Dente:** Pasta cooked to be firm when bitten.

29. **Beta-Carotene:** A precursor to vitamin A found in orange and dark green vegetables.

30. **Celiac Disease:** An autoimmune disorder triggered by gluten consumption.

31. **Dextrose:** A form of glucose often used as a sweetener.

32. **Emesis:** Vomiting or the act of expelling stomach contents.

33. **Fermentation:** The process of breaking down food by microorganisms, often used in food preservation.

34. **Ghee:** Clarified butter commonly used in Indian cuisine.

35. **Hemiplegia**: Paralysis affecting one side of the body.

36. **Infusion Pump:** Device for administering fluids or medications through a catheter.

37. **Jugular:** Pertaining to the large veins in the neck.

38. **Ketoacidosis:** A serious complication of diabetes characterized by high ketone levels.

39. **Lactose Intolerance:** Inability to digest lactose, a sugar in milk.

40. **Mediterranean Diet:** A diet inspired by the traditional eating patterns of countries bordering the Mediterranean Sea.

41. **NPO:** Nothing by mouth, indicating a temporary restriction from eating or drinking.

42. **Osteoporosis**: Condition characterized by weak and brittle bones.

43. **Palate:** The roof of the mouth, separating the oral and nasal cavities.

44. **Quinoa:** A nutrient-rich seed often used as a grain substitute.

45. **Roux:** A mixture of fat and flour used as a thickening agent in sauces.

46. **Sauté:** Cooking food quickly in a small amount of oil over high heat.

47. **Tachycardia:** Abnormally rapid heart rate.

48. **Umami:** A savory taste often associated with broths and cooked meats.

49. **Vegetarianism:** A diet excluding meat but including plant-based foods.

50. **Whole Foods:** Unprocessed or minimally processed foods in their natural state.

Dear Reader,

Thank you for choosing "Dysphagia Cookbook for Newly Diagnosed." Your commitment to exploring this resource reflects a dedication to health and well-being. I trust that the dysphagia-friendly recipes and insights within will serve as a valuable companion on your journey to flavorful and nourishing meals. Happy cooking and savoring every bite!

All the Best,

Emily O. Wells

www.ingramcontent.com/pod-product-compliance
Lightning Source LLC
Chambersburg PA
CBHW070821280726
48660CB00017B/2306